GLUTEN
NOT INCLUDED

*Your Complete Blueprint for
Navigating a Gluten-Free Lifestyle
with Confidence and Health*

VITA KRAUSE

clarifying purposes only and are owned by the owners themselves, not affiliated with this document.

TABLE OF CONTENTS

Chapter 1: The Gluten Basics

Understanding Gluten and Its Role in Modern Diets

Gluten, a protein found in wheat, barley, and rye, has become a topic of much debate and discussion in recent years. For some, it's a harmless component of their daily bread and pasta dishes. For others, it's a hidden culprit that can wreak havoc on their health. In this chapter, we'll delve into the world of gluten, exploring its origins, prevalence, and potential impact on our bodies.

The Gluten Conundrum

Once upon a time, gluten was just another protein, quietly present in the grains that have sustained civilizations for centuries. However, with the rise of industrialized food production and the widespread use of wheat in everything from bread to pasta to cereals, our exposure to gluten has skyrocketed.

Imagine a world where every meal, every snack, and even some beverages contain traces of this ubiquitous protein. It's no wonder that for those with sensitivities or intolerances, gluten can become a formidable foe.

The Gluten-Free Movement

As awareness of gluten-related disorders and sensitivities has grown, so too has the demand for gluten-free alternatives. No longer confined to the fringes of specialty stores, gluten-free options now grace the shelves of mainstream supermarkets, restaurants, and even fast-food chains.

This movement has been a blessing for those who must strictly avoid gluten, but it has also sparked a broader conversation about the role of gluten in our diets and its potential impact on our overall health.

The Science Behind Gluten

At its core, gluten is a protein composite found in wheat, barley, and rye. It's what gives bread its chewy texture and helps baked goods maintain their shape.

However, for individuals with conditions like celiac disease, an autoimmune disorder, consuming gluten can trigger a severe immune response that damages the small intestine.

Even for those without a diagnosed gluten-related disorder, some experts suggest that gluten may contribute to inflammation, digestive issues, and other health concerns in certain individuals.

Finding Your Gluten Balance

As with many aspects of nutrition and wellness, the impact of gluten on your body is highly individualized. Some people may have no issues with gluten whatsoever, while others may experience a range of symptoms, from mild discomfort to severe reactions.

The key is to listen to your body and work closely with healthcare professionals to determine if a gluten-free diet is right for you. Remember, a gluten-free lifestyle isn't a one-size-fits-all solution, but rather a personalized approach to optimizing your health and well-being.

In the chapters ahead, we'll dive deeper into the practical aspects of navigating a gluten-free lifestyle, exploring everything from reading labels and identifying hidden sources of gluten to creating delicious and satisfying gluten-free meals.

Signs and Symptoms of Gluten Sensitivity and Celiac Disease

Celiac disease is an autoimmune disorder that affects approximately 1% of the population. When individuals with celiac disease consume gluten, their immune system launches an attack on the small intestine, causing inflammation and damage to the villi – the tiny, fingerlike projections that line the intestine and absorb nutrients.

Common symptoms of celiac disease include:

- Chronic diarrhea or constipation

- Abdominal pain and bloating

- Fatigue and weakness

- Unexplained weight loss

- Anemia

- Bone or joint pain

- Skin rashes

It's crucial to note that celiac disease can present differently in children and adults, and some individuals may experience only mild or atypical symptoms, making diagnosis challenging.

Non-Celiac Gluten Sensitivity

While celiac disease is a well-defined autoimmune condition, there is a growing recognition of non-celiac gluten sensitivity (NCGS). Individuals with NCGS experience adverse reactions to gluten, despite testing negative for celiac disease and wheat allergy.

Symptoms of NCGS can mimic those of celiac disease, including:

- Digestive issues (bloating, gas, diarrhea, constipation)

- Headaches and migraines

- Fatigue and brain fog

- Joint and muscle pain

- Skin rashes or eczema

The exact cause of NCGS is not yet fully understood, but it is believed to involve an immune response or sensitivity to gluten or other components in wheat and related grains.

The Importance of Diagnosis

If you suspect that you may have celiac disease or a gluten sensitivity, it's crucial to seek proper medical attention and testing. Self-diagnosis can be dangerous, as it may lead to unnecessary dietary restrictions or delay treatment for other underlying conditions.

Your healthcare provider can order blood tests to screen for celiac disease and may recommend additional diagnostic procedures, such as an endoscopy or biopsy, if necessary.

Remember, while a gluten-free diet can alleviate symptoms for those with gluten-related disorders, it should not be adopted lightly or without proper guidance, as it can potentially lead to nutritional deficiencies if not implemented correctly.

The Science Behind Gluten-Related Disorders
Unraveling Celiac Disease

Celiac disease is an autoimmune disorder that occurs when the body's immune system mistakenly identifies gluten – a protein found in wheat, barley, and rye – as a threat. This triggers an inflammatory response that damages the small intestine, specifically the tiny, fingerlike projections called villi.

Picture these villi as the gatekeepers of nutrient absorption. When they become damaged, essential nutrients like iron, calcium, and vitamins struggle to pass through, leading to a wide range of potential symptoms and complications.

The Genetic Connection

Researchers have discovered that celiac disease has a strong genetic component. Individuals with certain genetic variations, particularly in the HLA-DQ2 and HLA-DQ8 genes, are more susceptible to developing the condition.

However, having these genetic markers doesn't necessarily mean you'll develop celiac disease. Environmental factors, such as exposure to gluten at an early age, infections, and gut health, also play a crucial role in triggering the autoimmune response.

Non-Celiac Gluten Sensitivity: A Puzzling Enigma

While celiac disease has a well-defined diagnostic criteria, non-celiac gluten sensitivity (NCGS) remains a bit of a mystery. Individuals with NCGS experience adverse reactions to gluten despite testing negative for celiac disease and wheat allergy.

The symptoms of NCGS can mimic those of celiac disease, including digestive issues, headaches, fatigue, and joint pain. However, unlike celiac disease, NCGS does not involve an autoimmune response or intestinal damage.

Researchers are still working to unravel the mechanisms behind NCGS, with theories ranging from immune system dysregulation to increased intestinal permeability (also known as "leaky gut").

The Wheat Protein Puzzle

Gluten isn't the only potential culprit when it comes to adverse reactions to wheat and related grains. Scientists are also investigating the role of other wheat proteins, such as amylase-trypsin inhibitors (ATIs) and fermentable oligo-, di-, monosaccharides, and polyols (FODMAPs).

These components may contribute to inflammation, digestive issues, and other symptoms in some individuals, even in the absence of gluten sensitivity or celiac disease.

A Journey of Self-Discovery

As you embark on your gluten-free journey, remember that every individual's experience with gluten-related disorders is unique. While understanding the science behind these conditions is crucial, it's equally important to listen to your body and work closely with healthcare professionals to determine the best course of action.

CHAPTER 2: THE DIAGNOSIS JOURNEY

Getting Tested for Gluten Sensitivity and Celiac Disease

Before you consider eliminating gluten from your diet, it's crucial to undergo proper testing. Self-diagnosing and initiating a gluten-free diet without medical guidance can lead to unnecessary dietary restrictions or delay the identification of other underlying conditions.

Furthermore, if you have celiac disease and start a gluten-free diet before being tested, it can lead to inaccurate test results, making it more challenging to receive an accurate diagnosis.

Testing for Celiac Disease

Celiac disease is an autoimmune disorder that can be diagnosed through a combination of blood tests and, in some cases, a biopsy of the small intestine.

Blood Tests

The first step in testing for celiac disease typically involves a blood test to check for specific antibodies that are produced when the immune system reacts to gluten. These tests include:

- Tissue Transglutaminase Antibodies (tTG-IgA)

- Endomysial Antibodies (EMA)

- Deamidated Gliadin Peptide Antibodies (DGP)

If the results of these blood tests are positive, your healthcare provider may recommend further testing or refer you to a gastroenterologist for additional evaluation.

Endoscopic Biopsy

In some cases, your doctor may recommend an endoscopic biopsy of the small intestine. During this procedure, a small sample of intestinal tissue is taken and examined for damage to the villi, which are the tiny, fingerlike projections that line the intestine and absorb nutrients.

Damage to the villi is a hallmark of celiac disease and can confirm the diagnosis.

Testing for Non-Celiac Gluten Sensitivity

Unlike celiac disease, there is no definitive test for non-celiac gluten sensitivity (NCGS). Instead, your healthcare provider may recommend an elimination diet, where you remove gluten from your diet for a period of time and monitor for improvement in symptoms.

If your symptoms improve after eliminating gluten and return when you reintroduce it, it may indicate a sensitivity or intolerance to gluten or other components in wheat and related grains.

Working with Your Healthcare Team

Throughout the testing process, it's essential to work closely with your healthcare team, which may include your primary care physician, a gastroenterologist, and a registered dietitian.

Be open and honest about your symptoms, medical history, and any concerns you may have. Your healthcare providers can help interpret test results, provide guidance on dietary modifications, and monitor your progress.

Remember, getting tested is just the first step on your gluten-free journey. In the chapters ahead, we'll explore practical strategies for navigating a gluten-free lifestyle, from reading labels and identifying hidden sources of gluten to creating delicious and nutritious meals that cater to your specific needs.

Interpreting Results and Next Steps
Positive for Celiac Disease

If your test results indicate that you have celiac disease, it's important to understand that this is a lifelong autoimmune disorder that requires strict adherence to a gluten-free diet. Upon receiving a positive diagnosis, you may experience a range of emotions, from relief at finally having an answer to apprehension about the dietary changes ahead.

Here are some key steps to take:

1. **Consult with a Gastroenterologist**: Work closely with a gastroenterologist who specializes in celiac disease. They can provide guidance on managing the condition, monitoring for potential complications, and ensuring proper nutrient absorption.

2. **Meet with a Registered Dietitian**: A registered dietitian with expertise in celiac disease can help you navigate the gluten-free diet, ensuring you're getting adequate nutrition and avoiding hidden sources of gluten.

3. **Join Support Groups**: Connecting with others who are living with celiac disease can be incredibly valuable. Support groups offer a sense of community, shared experiences, and practical tips for maintaining a gluten-free lifestyle.

4. **Educate Yourself**: Knowledge is power when it comes to managing celiac disease. Take the time to learn about gluten-free food labeling, cross-contamination risks, and how to adapt your favorite recipes to be gluten-free.

Negative for Celiac Disease, but Positive for Non-Celiac Gluten Sensitivity

If your test results are negative for celiac disease but you experience improvements in symptoms after eliminating gluten, you may have non-celiac gluten sensitivity (NCGS). This condition is not as well-understood as celiac disease, but it still requires careful management of your diet.

Steps to consider include:

1. **Work with a Registered Dietitian**: A dietitian can help you navigate the gluten-free diet and ensure you're meeting your nutritional needs.

2. **Monitor Symptom Improvement**: Keep a food journal and track any changes in your symptoms

after eliminating gluten. This can help you determine the extent of your sensitivity.

3. **Explore Other Potential Triggers**: In some cases, NCGS may be related to sensitivity to other components in wheat or grains, such as FODMAPs or amylase-trypsin inhibitors (ATIs). Your healthcare provider may recommend additional testing or dietary modifications.

4. **Be Mindful of Cross-Contamination**: While your sensitivity may not be as severe as celiac disease, it's still important to avoid cross-contamination with gluten to manage your symptoms effectively.

Negative for Both Celiac Disease and Non-Celiac Gluten Sensitivity

If your test results are negative for both celiac disease and non-celiac gluten sensitivity, but you still experience persistent symptoms, it's important to continue working with your healthcare team to identify the underlying cause.

Potential next steps may include:

1. **Exploring Other Food Sensitivities or Intolerances**: Your symptoms may be related to sensitivity to other foods or components, such as dairy, soy, or FODMAPs.

2. **Investigating Digestive Disorders**: Conditions like irritable bowel syndrome (IBS), inflammatory bowel disease (IBD), or small intestinal bacterial overgrowth (SIBO) can sometimes mimic symptoms associated with gluten sensitivity.

3. **Considering Other Medical Conditions**: Persistent symptoms may also be related to other medical conditions, such as thyroid disorders, anemia, or autoimmune diseases.

4. **Seeking Additional Testing or Specialist Referrals**: Your healthcare provider may

recommend additional testing or referrals to specialists, such as gastroenterologists, allergists, or nutritionists, to further investigate your symptoms.

Remember, interpreting test results and determining the appropriate next steps is a collaborative process between you and your healthcare team. Open communication, patience, and a willingness to explore various avenues are key to finding the right path forward.

Emotional and Psychological Aspects of a Gluten Diagnosis

A gluten-related diagnosis can trigger a whirlwind of emotions, ranging from relief at finally having an explanation for your symptoms to anxiety about the dietary and lifestyle changes that lie ahead. It's perfectly normal to experience a myriad of feelings, including:

- **Grief**: You may mourn the loss of your previous dietary freedom and the need to bid farewell to certain beloved foods or traditions.

- **Overwhelm**: The prospect of overhauling your diet and lifestyle can feel daunting, especially in the beginning stages.

- **Frustration**: Navigating social situations, dining out, and reading labels can be frustrating and may evoke feelings of isolation or resentment.

- **Fear**: Concerns about cross-contamination, potential health complications, or the long-term impact on your quality of life may arise.

- **Relief**: For some, finally receiving a diagnosis can bring a sense of validation and relief, providing answers to long-standing health issues.

It's essential to acknowledge and process these emotions, as they are natural and valid responses to a significant life change.

Coping Strategies and Support Systems

Navigating the emotional and psychological aspects of a gluten-related diagnosis can be challenging, but there are strategies and support systems that can help you along the way:

1. **Seek Professional Support**: Don't hesitate to reach out to a therapist, counselor, or support group facilitator to help you process the emotional impact of your diagnosis and develop coping mechanisms.

2. **Build a Support Network**: Surround yourself with understanding friends, family members, or online communities who can offer encouragement, practical advice, and a listening ear.

3. **Practice Self-Compassion**: Be kind and patient with yourself as you navigate this new terrain. Celebrate small victories and acknowledge the challenges without harsh self-judgment.

4. **Find Gluten-Free Role Models**: Connect with individuals who have successfully embraced a gluten-free lifestyle and learn from their experiences and insights.

5. **Develop Stress Management Techniques**: Incorporate stress-relieving practices, such as mindfulness, exercise, or hobbies, to help you cope with the emotional demands of your new reality.

6. **Reframe Your Perspective**: Instead of viewing your diagnosis as a limitation, embrace it as an opportunity to prioritize your health and explore new culinary adventures.

Remember, the emotional and psychological journey is just as important as the physical one. By cultivating self-compassion, seeking support, and embracing coping strategies, you can navigate this transition with greater resilience and a renewed sense of empowerment.

CHAPTER 3: SETTING UP YOUR GLUTEN-FREE KITCHEN

Essential Gluten-Free Pantry Staples

Gluten-Free Flours: The Foundation of Your Baking Empire

Baking without wheat flour may seem like a daunting task, but fear not, for the gluten-free realm offers a plethora of delightful alternatives. Here are some must-have flours to stock your pantry:

- **Almond Flour**: Nutrient-dense and deliciously nutty, almond flour lends a rich texture to baked goods.

- **Rice Flour**: Available in both white and brown varieties, rice flour is a versatile and mild-tasting option.

- **Coconut Flour**: With its unique properties and subtle coconut flavor, this flour adds moisture and tenderness to your creations.

- **Oat Flour**: Ensure you choose certified gluten-free oat flour, as regular oats can be cross-contaminated with gluten.

- **Tapioca Flour**: A staple for its binding properties and ability to create a light and airy texture.

Pro Tip: Experiment with blending different flours to achieve the perfect texture and flavor for your desired baked goods.

Grains and Starches: The Gluten-Free Carb Crew

Bid farewell to wheat-based pastas and breads, and embrace the diverse world of gluten-free grains and starches:

- **Quinoa**: A nutritional powerhouse packed with protein, fiber, and a nutty flavor.

- **Buckwheat Groats**: Despite the name, buckwheat is naturally gluten-free and offers a hearty, earthy taste.

- **Cornmeal and Polenta**: Versatile ingredients perfect for everything from cornbread to polenta fries.

- **Potato Starch and Arrowroot Powder**: Invaluable for thickening sauces and adding structure to baked goods.

Condiments and Seasonings: Flavor Boosters Extraordinaire

Bid adieu to bland and tasteless meals! These gluten-free condiments and seasonings will elevate your culinary creations to new heights:

- **Tamari or Coconut Aminos**: Gluten-free alternatives to soy sauce, adding depth and umami to dishes.

- **Gluten-Free Broth or Stock**: Indispensable for soups, stews, and sauces, with a variety of flavors to choose from.

- **Herbs and Spices**: Experiment with fresh and dried herbs, spice blends, and seasonings to add layers of flavor to your meals.

- **Vinegars**: From balsamic to apple cider, vinegars can brighten and balance flavors in dressings and marinades.

Pantry Essentials: The Gluten-Free MVPs

Round out your pantry with these versatile and trusty staples:

- **Gluten-Free Oats**: Certified gluten-free oats can be enjoyed for breakfast, baking, and more.

- **Nuts and Seeds**: From almonds to chia seeds, these nutrient-dense additions offer crunch, protein, and healthy fats.

- **Gluten-Free Crackers and Snacks**: For those moments when a quick bite is needed, keep a stash of tasty gluten-free options on hand.

☐ **Canned Goods**: Stock up on gluten-free canned beans, tomatoes, and broths for quick and easy meal prep.

Remember, a well-stocked gluten-free pantry is the foundation for a diverse and delicious gluten-free lifestyle. Experiment, explore, and don't be afraid to venture beyond the familiar – the possibilities are endless!

Cross-Contamination: What to Watch For
Understanding Cross-Contamination

Cross-contamination occurs when gluten-containing foods come into contact with gluten-free foods, either through direct contact or by sharing utensils, cooking surfaces, or equipment. Even minuscule amounts of gluten can trigger adverse reactions in individuals with celiac disease or severe gluten sensitivity, making cross-contamination a serious concern.

Common Sources of Cross-Contamination

Cross-contamination can happen in various settings, including:

1. **Kitchen Surfaces and Utensils**: Cutting boards, countertops, knives, and other cooking utensils can harbor gluten residue if not properly cleaned after handling gluten-containing foods.

2. **Shared Condiments and Spreads**: Double-dipping utensils or using the same container for gluten-free and gluten-containing items can lead to cross-contamination.

3. **Deep Fryers and Shared Cooking Oils**: If a deep fryer or cooking oil has been used for gluten-containing foods, it can inadvertently contaminate gluten-free items cooked in the same oil.

4. **Restaurants and Food Service Establishments**: Cross-contamination can occur in restaurant kitchens if proper protocols are not followed, such as using dedicated cooking

surfaces, utensils, and preparation areas for gluten-free items.

5. **Shared Living Spaces**: In households where both gluten-free and gluten-containing foods are present, cross-contamination can occur if proper precautions are not taken.

Strategies to Prevent Cross-Contamination

While cross-contamination can be a daunting concern, there are several practical strategies you can employ to minimize the risk:

1. **Dedicate Cooking Utensils and Surfaces**: Invest in separate cutting boards, knives, and cooking utensils specifically for gluten-free food preparation. Clearly label them to avoid confusion.

2. **Clean Thoroughly**: Always clean cooking surfaces, utensils, and appliances thoroughly before and after handling gluten-free foods. Use

dedicated sponges or cloths to avoid cross-contact with gluten residue.

3. **Separate Storage**: Store gluten-free foods in designated areas, separate from gluten-containing items, to prevent accidental mixing or spillage.

4. **Restaurant Awareness**: When dining out, communicate your dietary needs clearly to restaurant staff and inquire about their cross-contamination prevention protocols.

5. **Educate Household Members**: If you share a living space, educate other household members about the importance of avoiding cross-contamination and establish designated gluten-free zones in the kitchen.

6. **Label and Color-Code**: Use labels or color-coding systems to clearly identify gluten-free items, utensils, and cooking surfaces, making it easier to avoid mistakes.

Remember, even the smallest trace of gluten can have severe consequences for those with celiac disease or severe gluten sensitivity. By staying vigilant, implementing practical strategies, and educating those around you, you can significantly reduce the risk of cross-contamination and enjoy a safe and healthy gluten-free lifestyle.

Shopping for Gluten-Free Products: Label Reading 101

Understanding Gluten-Free Labeling

The first step in deciphering labels is to familiarize yourself with the terminology and regulations surrounding gluten-free claims. According to the Food and Drug Administration (FDA), a product can be labeled "gluten-free" if it contains less than 20 parts per million (ppm) of gluten, a level considered safe for most individuals with celiac disease or gluten sensitivity.

However, it's important to note that not all products are required to carry a "gluten-free" label, even if they meet the criteria. This is where your label reading skills become invaluable.

Decoding Ingredients Lists

The ingredients list is your ultimate guide to uncovering hidden sources of gluten. Here are some key things to look for:

1. **Wheat and Wheat Derivatives**: Avoid products containing wheat, wheat flour, wheat gluten, wheat starch, and other wheat-derived ingredients.

2. **Barley and Rye**: These grains, along with their derivatives, must also be avoided as they contain gluten.

3. **Ambiguous Ingredients**: Be cautious of ingredients like "modified food starch," "natural flavors," or "malt" – these can potentially contain gluten unless explicitly labeled as gluten-free.

4. **Certified Gluten-Free Labels**: Look for products with a "Certified Gluten-Free" seal from reputable organizations, as this provides an extra layer of assurance that the product meets strict gluten-free standards.

Reading Between the Lines

While ingredients lists are invaluable, there are other aspects of label reading that can help you navigate the gluten-free landscape:

1. **Cross-Contamination Statements**: Some products may carry a "may contain" or "processed in a facility" statement, indicating a risk of cross-contamination with gluten-containing ingredients.

2. **Allergen Statements**: Products that contain wheat or other gluten-containing grains as an allergen will typically be clearly labeled as such.

3. **Imported Products**: Be aware that imported products may not adhere to the same gluten-free

labeling regulations as domestic products, so extra caution is advised.

Building Confidence in Label Reading

Becoming a proficient label reader takes time and practice, but with each shopping trip, your confidence and expertise will grow. Don't be afraid to ask questions, research unfamiliar ingredients, and consult with healthcare professionals or support groups if you're unsure about a product's gluten-free status.

Remember, the power to make informed choices lies in your hands, and by mastering the art of label reading, you'll be able to navigate the grocery aisles with ease, ensuring that every item in your cart aligns with your gluten-free lifestyle.

CHAPTER 4: THE ART OF GLUTEN-FREE COOKING

Basic Gluten-Free Cooking Techniques

Baking without gluten can be a daunting prospect, but with the right techniques and ingredients, you'll soon be whipping up treats that rival their gluten-filled counterparts. Here are some essential tips to get you started:

1. **Flour Blends**: Experiment with different gluten-free flour blends to find the perfect combination for your desired texture and flavor. Popular options include rice flour, almond flour, and tapioca starch.

2. **Binding Agents**: Gluten-free baked goods often require additional binding agents to hold their shape, such as xanthan gum, psyllium husk, or ground flaxseed.

3. **Leavening**: Ensure your baking powder and baking soda are gluten-free, and consider adding extra leavening agents like egg whites or vinegar for a light, airy texture.

4. **Moisture Management**: Gluten-free baked goods tend to dry out faster, so adjust baking times and temperatures as needed, and consider adding moisture-rich ingredients like applesauce or yogurt.

Mastering Gluten-Free Cooking

Beyond baking, there are several techniques and substitutions that will elevate your gluten-free cooking game:

1. **Thickening Agents**: Instead of wheat flour for thickening sauces and gravies, reach for gluten-free alternatives like cornstarch, arrowroot powder, or tapioca starch.

2. **Breadcrumbs and Coatings**: For crispy coatings or breadcrumb toppings, grind up

gluten-free crackers, nuts, or certified gluten-free breadcrumbs.

3. **Gluten-Free Grains and Pastas**: Explore the world of gluten-free grains like quinoa, amaranth, and buckwheat, as well as gluten-free pasta options made from rice, corn, or legumes.

4. **Gluten-Free Flours for Roux and Dredging**: Instead of wheat flour, use gluten-free alternatives like rice flour, cornstarch, or tapioca starch for making roux or dredging proteins.

Kitchen Safety and Cross-Contamination Prevention

As you delve into gluten-free cooking, it's essential to maintain a safe and contamination-free environment. Dedicate separate cooking utensils, cutting boards, and preparation surfaces for gluten-free foods, and ensure thorough cleaning to avoid cross-contact with gluten-containing ingredients.

Remember, the key to success in the gluten-free kitchen lies in experimentation, patience, and a willingness to adapt traditional techniques to suit your dietary needs. Embrace the adventure, and soon you'll be creating culinary masterpieces that not only satisfy your taste buds but also nourish your body and soul.

Transforming Your Favorite Recipes
Understanding Gluten's Role in Recipes

Before diving into recipe transformation, it's important to understand the role gluten plays in traditional recipes. Gluten, a protein found in wheat, rye, and barley, acts as a binding agent, providing structure and elasticity to baked goods, breads, and more. When removing gluten, it's essential to find suitable replacements that can mimic these properties and maintain the desired texture and consistency.

Ingredient Substitutions and Replacements

One of the keys to successful recipe transformation lies in mastering ingredient substitutions and replacements. Here are some essential swaps to consider:

1. **Flours**: Swap wheat flour for gluten-free alternatives like almond flour, rice flour, or a gluten-free all-purpose flour blend.

2. **Binding Agents**: Replace gluten with alternative binders like xanthan gum, psyllium husk, or ground flaxseed to help maintain structure.

3. **Breadcrumbs and Coatings**: Instead of traditional breadcrumbs, use crushed gluten-free crackers, nuts, or certified gluten-free breadcrumbs.

4. **Thickeners**: Swap wheat flour for gluten-free thickeners like cornstarch, arrowroot powder, or tapioca starch when making roux, gravies, or sauces.

5. **Grains and Pastas**: Substitute wheat-based grains and pastas with gluten-free alternatives

like quinoa, amaranth, or gluten-free pasta made from rice, corn, or legumes.

Adapting Techniques and Methods

In addition to ingredient substitutions, you may need to adapt cooking techniques and methods to ensure success with your transformed recipes. Here are some tips to keep in mind:

1. **Baking Times and Temperatures**: Gluten-free baked goods often require adjustments to baking times and temperatures due to differences in moisture absorption and density.

2. **Mixing and Kneading**: Gluten-free doughs and batters may require less mixing or kneading to prevent over-developing the structure.

3. **Moisture Management**: Gluten-free baked goods tend to dry out faster, so consider adding moisture-rich ingredients like applesauce, yogurt, or additional eggs.

4. **Leavening Agents**: Adjust the amount of leavening agents like baking powder, baking soda, or egg whites to achieve the desired rise and texture.

Embracing Experimentation and Patience

Transforming beloved recipes is an art that requires experimentation, patience, and a willingness to adapt. Don't be discouraged if your first attempts aren't perfect – treat each attempt as a learning experience and make adjustments as needed. Consider keeping a recipe notebook to track your successes and challenges, and don't be afraid to seek guidance from gluten-free cookbooks, online resources, or support groups.

Remember, the joy of transforming your favorite recipes lies not only in the delicious results but also in the process of preserving cherished traditions and flavors while honoring your dietary needs. Embrace the journey, celebrate your successes, and savor the memories that come with each bite.

Time-Saving Tips for Busy Lives
Batch Cooking and Meal Prepping

One of the most effective time-saving techniques is batch cooking and meal prepping. By dedicating a few hours on your day off or a quiet weekend, you can prepare a week's worth of gluten-free meals and snacks, saving you valuable time during the workweek. Here are some tips to get you started:

- **Invest in Quality Storage Containers**: Reusable, airtight containers are essential for storing prepped meals and ingredients.

- **Prepare Base Ingredients**: Cook grains, roast vegetables, and prepare proteins in bulk, then mix and match throughout the week.

- **Freeze Portions**: Freeze individual portions of soups, stews, or casseroles for a quick, hassle-free meal.

- **Plan Your Meals**: Create a weekly meal plan to streamline your shopping and prep efforts.

Embrace One-Pot and Sheet Pan Meals

One-pot and sheet pan meals are a gluten-free kitchen's best friend. Not only do they minimize cleanup, but they also allow you to cook an entire meal in one vessel or on a single pan. Consider recipes like:

- **Gluten-Free Stir-Fries**: Toss your choice of protein, vegetables, and a gluten-free sauce for a quick and flavorful meal.

- **Roasted Sheet Pan Meals**: Arrange proteins, vegetables, and seasonings on a sheet pan for a hands-off cooking experience.

- **Gluten-Free Casseroles**: Layer ingredients in a baking dish for a complete, hassle-free meal.

Stock Up on Gluten-Free Convenience Items

While homemade meals are often the healthiest option, there's no shame in relying on gluten-free convenience items to save time and effort. Keep your pantry stocked with items like:

- **Gluten-Free Frozen Meals**: Look for high-quality, gluten-free frozen meals or meal components for busy nights.

- **Pre-Cooked Proteins**: Rotisserie chickens, canned fish, or pre-cooked gluten-free sausages can be a quick protein source.

- **Gluten-Free Snacks**: Keep a selection of gluten-free snacks on hand for on-the-go fuel.

Utilize Time-Saving Kitchen Gadgets

Invest in a few key kitchen gadgets to streamline your gluten-free cooking routine:

- **Slow Cooker or Instant Pot**: These versatile appliances allow you to prepare hands-off meals with minimal effort.

- **High-Powered Blender**: Quickly whip up gluten-free smoothies, soups, or sauces.

- **Food Processor**: Chop, grate, and shred ingredients in a fraction of the time.

Remember, the key to successful time management in the gluten-free kitchen is finding a balance between convenience and nourishment. By implementing these time-saving strategies, you'll be able to enjoy delicious, gluten-free meals without sacrificing precious hours in the kitchen.

Chapter 5: Navigating Social Situations

Eating Out and Staying Gluten-Free

Researching and Planning Ahead

Before venturing out, take the time to research gluten-free-friendly restaurants in your area. Many establishments now offer dedicated gluten-free menus or clearly mark gluten-free options, making it easier to make informed choices. Additionally, consult online reviews, restaurant websites, and gluten-free dining guides to gain insights into establishments with a proven track record of accommodating dietary restrictions.

Communicating Your Needs

Clear and effective communication with restaurant staff is crucial when dining out gluten-free. When ordering, be specific about your dietary needs and don't hesitate to ask questions about ingredients, preparation methods, and cross-contamination protocols. Some key phrases to keep in mind:

- "I have a gluten allergy/sensitivity, and I need to avoid any exposure to gluten."

- "Can you please confirm that this dish is completely gluten-free, including any sauces or seasonings?"

- "Can you ensure that dedicated gluten-free cooking surfaces and utensils are used for my order?"

Additionally, don't be afraid to politely request substitutions or modifications to ensure your meal is truly gluten-free.

Navigating Menus

When perusing restaurant menus, keep an eye out for dishes that are naturally gluten-free, such as grilled proteins, steamed or roasted vegetables, and salads (without croutons or gluten-containing dressings). Be cautious of dishes that may contain hidden sources of gluten, such as soups, sauces, and breaded or fried items.

If a gluten-free menu is not available, don't hesitate to ask your server for guidance or consult with the chef directly. Many establishments are now well-versed in accommodating gluten-free diners and can make appropriate adjustments to existing menu items.

Cross-Contamination Awareness

Cross-contamination is a significant concern when dining out, as even trace amounts of gluten can cause adverse reactions for those with celiac disease or severe gluten sensitivity. When ordering, inquire about the restaurant's cross-contamination prevention protocols, such as:

- Dedicated gluten-free cooking surfaces and utensils

- Proper storage and handling of gluten-free ingredients

☐ Staff training on gluten-free food preparation

Additionally, be cautious of shared fryers, shared condiment containers, and buffet or self-serve stations, which can increase the risk of cross-contamination.

Packing Gluten-Free Essentials

To ensure a smooth dining experience, consider packing a few gluten-free essentials in your bag or purse. This can include gluten-free snacks or bread in case of limited options, as well as a small card or information sheet explaining your dietary needs to show restaurant staff.

Remember, dining out while maintaining a gluten-free lifestyle is entirely possible with the right preparation, communication, and awareness. By following these strategies, you can enjoy the social and culinary experiences of eating out without compromising your health or dietary restrictions.

Communicating Your Needs Effectively

Building a Foundation of Knowledge

The first step in effective communication is arming yourself with knowledge about celiac disease, gluten sensitivity, and the gluten-free lifestyle. Educate yourself on the potential health risks associated with gluten exposure, the importance of avoiding cross-contamination, and the various sources of gluten in foods and products. This knowledge will not only help you make informed choices but also empower you to articulate your needs clearly and confidently to others.

Navigating Social Situations

Social gatherings, such as parties, potlucks, or family events, can be a minefield for those following a gluten-free diet. To navigate these situations successfully, consider the following strategies:

1. **Offer to Bring a Dish**: By bringing a gluten-free dish to share, you ensure there's at least one safe option available for you to enjoy.

2. **Communicate in Advance**: If possible, inform the host or organizer about your dietary needs ahead of time, allowing them to make appropriate accommodations.

3. **Educate with Empathy**: When explaining your dietary restrictions, approach the conversation with empathy and understanding. Avoid accusatory language or making others feel guilty for their lack of knowledge.

4. **Suggest Alternatives**: If a particular dish or activity involves gluten, offer gluten-free alternatives or suggestions to make the event more inclusive for you.

Dining Out with Confidence

Communicating your needs effectively when dining out is crucial for ensuring a safe and enjoyable experience. Here are some tips to keep in mind:

1. **Be Specific**: Clearly state that you have a gluten allergy or sensitivity, and request gluten-free

preparation methods and dedicated cooking surfaces.

2. **Ask Questions**: Don't be afraid to inquire about ingredients, cooking methods, and cross-contamination protocols. It's better to be thorough than to risk exposure.

3. **Provide Resources**: If the restaurant staff seems unfamiliar with gluten-free requirements, consider providing educational resources or offering to clarify any misunderstandings.

4. **Express Gratitude**: When your needs are accommodated, express your appreciation to the staff. Positive reinforcement can go a long way in fostering understanding and awareness.

Workplace and Professional Settings

Navigating dietary needs in the workplace can be challenging, but open communication and advocacy are key to creating an inclusive environment. Consider the following strategies:

1. **Inform Colleagues and Supervisors**: Share your dietary needs with your colleagues and supervisors, explaining the importance of avoiding gluten exposure.

2. **Request Accommodations**: For work-related events or meetings, request gluten-free meal options or the ability to bring your own food.

3. **Advocate for Awareness**: Suggest hosting a gluten-free awareness session or providing educational resources to promote understanding among your colleagues.

4. **Lead by Example**: By demonstrating professionalism and open communication, you can set a positive example for others to follow.

Remember, effective communication is not just about conveying information – it's about fostering understanding, building bridges, and creating an inclusive environment where your needs are respected and accommodated. By approaching conversations with empathy, knowledge, and confidence, you can navigate the gluten-free journey with ease and empower those around you to support your dietary choices.

Handling Social Pressure and Misunderstandings

Before addressing social pressure or misunderstandings, it's essential to recognize that they often stem from a lack of knowledge or awareness about celiac disease, gluten sensitivity, and the gluten-free lifestyle. Many people may have misconceptions or oversimplify the complexities of living gluten-free, leading to dismissive or unsupportive attitudes. By approaching these situations with empathy and understanding, you can create opportunities for education and foster a more inclusive environment.

Responding with Patience and Education

When faced with social pressure or misunderstandings, your first instinct may be to react defensively or with frustration. However, it's often more effective to respond with patience and a willingness to educate. Here are some strategies to consider:

1. **Remain Calm**: Take a deep breath and avoid reacting emotionally. Approach the situation with a level head and a desire to foster understanding.

2. **Share Your Story**: Explain your personal journey with celiac disease or gluten sensitivity, and the impact it has had on your health and well-being. Personal stories can be powerful tools for building empathy and understanding.

3. **Provide Resources**: Have a few reputable resources or informational materials on hand to share with those who may be unfamiliar with the gluten-free lifestyle. This can help reinforce the seriousness of your dietary needs.

4. **Offer Alternatives**: If social pressure arises around food or activities, suggest gluten-free

alternatives or compromises that allow you to participate without compromising your health.

5. **Lead by Example**: By maintaining a positive and respectful attitude, even in the face of misunderstandings, you can set an example for others to follow and foster a more inclusive environment.

Setting Boundaries and Prioritizing Self-Care

While education and open communication are essential, there may be situations where you need to set firm boundaries to protect your well-being. Remember, your health and safety should always be the top priority. Here are some strategies to consider:

1. **Politely Decline**: If a social situation or activity poses a significant risk of gluten exposure or makes you uncomfortable, feel empowered to politely decline without guilt or apology.

2. **Seek Support**: Lean on your support system, whether it's friends, family, or a gluten-free

community, to help you navigate challenging situations and provide emotional support.

3. **Practice Self-Care**: Engage in activities that promote your mental and emotional well-being, such as meditation, exercise, or pursuing hobbies that bring you joy and relaxation.

4. **Prioritize Your Needs**: Remind yourself that your dietary needs are valid and important, and that you have the right to prioritize your health without feeling guilty or pressured.

Remember, navigating social pressure and misunderstandings is an ongoing journey, and there may be setbacks or frustrating moments along the way. However, by approaching these situations with patience, education, and a commitment to self-care, you can build resilience and create a more inclusive and supportive environment for your gluten-free lifestyle.

CHAPTER 6: GLUTEN-FREE NUTRITION AND WELLNESS

Building a Balanced Gluten-Free Diet

Before diving into dietary planning, it's important to understand the key nutrients that should be prioritized in a gluten-free diet. Some essential nutrients to focus on include:

1. **Fiber**: With the elimination of many whole grains, it's essential to incorporate fiber-rich foods like fruits, vegetables, beans, and gluten-free whole grains.

2. **Iron**: Iron deficiency is common among those following a gluten-free diet, as many iron-rich foods like fortified breads and cereals are off-limits. Incorporate lean meats, leafy greens, and iron-fortified gluten-free products.

3. **B Vitamins**: Gluten-free grains are often not enriched with B vitamins like thiamine,

riboflavin, niacin, and folate, which are essential for energy production and overall health.

4. **Calcium and Vitamin D**: With the absence of fortified dairy products in some gluten-free diets, it's crucial to focus on calcium and vitamin D-rich foods or consider supplementation.

Building a Balanced Plate

One of the simplest ways to ensure a balanced gluten-free diet is to follow the principles of a balanced plate. This approach involves incorporating a variety of nutrient-dense foods from each food group at every meal:

1. **Proteins**: Lean meats, poultry, fish, eggs, legumes, and soy-based products provide essential amino acids and nutrients.

2. **Fruits and Vegetables**: Aim for a colorful variety of fresh, frozen, or canned fruits and veggies to ensure a wide range of vitamins, minerals, and antioxidants.

3. **Gluten-Free Grains and Starches**: Quinoa, brown rice, amaranth, and gluten-free oats are excellent sources of complex carbohydrates, fiber, and various micronutrients.

4. **Healthy Fats**: Incorporate healthy fats like avocados, nuts, seeds, and olive oil for essential fatty acids and nutrient absorption.

5. **Dairy or Dairy Alternatives**: If tolerated, include low-fat dairy products or fortified plant-based alternatives for calcium, vitamin D, and protein.

Meal Planning and Preparation

Proper meal planning and preparation can make a big difference in maintaining a balanced gluten-free diet. Consider the following strategies:

1. **Create a Weekly Meal Plan**: Plan out your meals and snacks for the week, ensuring a variety of nutrient-dense foods and minimizing the temptation of less healthful choices.

2. **Batch Cook and Meal Prep**: Dedicate time on weekends or free evenings to batch cook and meal prep, making it easier to have nutritious options on hand.

3. **Stock Up on Gluten-Free Pantry Staples**: Keep your kitchen stocked with gluten-free grains, beans, lentils, canned fish, and other nutrient-dense staples for quick meal assembly.

4. **Experiment with New Recipes**: Explore new gluten-free recipes and cuisines to keep your diet interesting and varied, ensuring you're exposed to a wide range of nutrients.

Remember, building a balanced gluten-free diet is not about deprivation or restriction – it's about embracing a variety of delicious and nourishing foods that support your overall health and well-being. By focusing on nutrient-dense choices, proper meal planning, and variety, you can thrive on a gluten-free diet while enjoying every bite.

Supplements and Nutrients of Concern

Several nutrients have been identified as being at a higher risk of deficiency in individuals following a gluten-free diet. It's essential to be aware of these nutrients and take steps to ensure adequate intake through dietary sources or supplementation.

1. **Fiber**: Many gluten-free products are made from refined grains, which are lower in fiber than their whole-grain counterparts. Inadequate fiber intake can lead to digestive issues and an increased risk of chronic diseases.

2. **Iron**: Gluten-free diets often lack fortified grains, which are a significant source of iron in traditional diets. Iron deficiency can lead to fatigue, weakness, and impaired immune function.

3. **Folate (Vitamin B9)**: Fortified grains are a major source of folate, which is essential for red blood

cell production and preventing neural tube defects during pregnancy.

4. **Vitamin B12**: While not directly related to gluten, some individuals following a gluten-free diet may also restrict animal products, increasing the risk of vitamin B12 deficiency.

5. **Calcium and Vitamin D**: Dairy products are a significant source of calcium and vitamin D, and individuals avoiding gluten may also limit dairy intake, increasing the risk of deficiency.

6. **Zinc**: Whole grains and fortified cereals are good sources of zinc, which is essential for immune function, wound healing, and growth.

The Role of Supplements

While it's always preferable to obtain nutrients from whole, nutrient-dense foods, supplements can play a crucial role in bridging any nutritional gaps in a gluten-free diet. However, it's important to consult with a healthcare professional or registered dietitian before starting any supplement regimen, as excessive or unnecessary supplementation can have potential risks.

1. **Multivitamin/Mineral Supplement**: A gluten-free multivitamin/mineral supplement can help ensure adequate intake of essential nutrients, particularly those identified as being at risk of deficiency.

2. **Targeted Supplements**: Based on individual needs or deficiencies, targeted supplements such as iron, folate, vitamin B12, calcium, or zinc may be recommended.

3. **Fiber Supplements**: If dietary fiber intake remains low despite efforts to include more fiber-rich foods, a fiber supplement may be beneficial for maintaining proper digestive health.

4. **Probiotics**: Individuals with celiac disease or gluten sensitivity may benefit from probiotic supplements to support gut health and improve nutrient absorption.

It's important to note that supplements should never be used as a substitute for a balanced, nutrient-dense diet. Instead, they should be viewed as a complement to a well-planned gluten-free eating plan, helping to fill any remaining nutritional gaps and support overall health and well-being.

Remember, the key to a successful gluten-free lifestyle is not just about avoiding gluten but also about nourishing your body with a variety of nutrient-rich foods and addressing any potential deficiencies through appropriate supplementation when necessary.

The Impact of Gluten-Free Living on Overall Health

For those with celiac disease or gluten sensitivity, the removal of gluten from the diet can have a profound impact on digestive health. Gluten can trigger an autoimmune response in individuals with celiac disease, leading to inflammation and damage to the small intestine. By eliminating gluten, the intestinal lining can heal, allowing for improved nutrient absorption and alleviation of symptoms such as bloating, diarrhea, constipation, and abdominal pain.

Even for those without diagnosed gluten-related conditions, a gluten-free diet may promote better digestive health by reducing inflammation and improving gut microbiome balance.

Reduced Inflammation and Autoimmune Regulation

Gluten has been linked to increased inflammation throughout the body, which can contribute to a variety of chronic health conditions, including autoimmune disorders. By removing gluten from the diet, many individuals experience a reduction in systemic inflammation, which can have far-reaching benefits for overall health.

For those with autoimmune conditions like rheumatoid arthritis, multiple sclerosis, or Hashimoto's thyroiditis, a gluten-free diet may help regulate the immune system's response, potentially reducing symptom severity and disease progression.

Improved Energy Levels and Mental Clarity

Brain fog, fatigue, and difficulty concentrating are common complaints among those with undiagnosed gluten sensitivity or celiac disease. When the body is constantly fighting inflammation and struggling to absorb nutrients properly, energy levels can plummet, and cognitive function can suffer.

By adopting a gluten-free lifestyle, many individuals report experiencing a significant improvement in energy levels, mental clarity, and overall cognitive function. This can be attributed to reduced inflammation, improved nutrient absorption, and the elimination of any potential neurotoxic effects of gluten on the brain.

Potential Weight Management Benefits

For some individuals, eliminating gluten may aid in weight management efforts. Gluten-containing foods, particularly those made with refined grains, can contribute to insulin resistance, inflammation, and hormonal imbalances, all of which can make weight loss more challenging.

By adopting a gluten-free diet focused on whole, nutrient-dense foods, many individuals experience improved satiety, better blood sugar regulation, and a reduction in inflammatory processes that can contribute to weight gain or difficulty losing weight.

Reduced Risk of Chronic Diseases

The benefits of a gluten-free lifestyle extend beyond symptom management for those with gluten-related disorders. By promoting better digestive health, reducing inflammation, and supporting overall nutrient absorption, a gluten-free diet may also play a role in reducing the risk of chronic diseases such as:

- Cardiovascular disease

- Type 2 diabetes

- Certain types of cancer

- Alzheimer's disease and dementia

While more research is needed to fully understand the potential preventive benefits of a gluten-free lifestyle, the evidence suggests that the reduction of inflammation and improved overall health can have a positive impact on chronic disease risk.

It's important to note that while a gluten-free lifestyle can be highly beneficial for many individuals, it's not a panacea or a cure-all solution. It's crucial to work closely with healthcare professionals, registered dietitians, and other experts to ensure that your dietary needs are met, and any underlying health conditions are properly managed.

Additionally, it's essential to recognize that a gluten-free diet alone is not a guarantee of good health – it's equally important to focus on consuming a balanced, nutrient-dense diet rich in whole, unprocessed foods, engaging in regular physical activity, and practicing stress management techniques.

By embracing a gluten-free lifestyle with a holistic approach, you can unlock the potential for improved overall health, increased energy levels, and a renewed sense of vitality, while also managing any gluten-related conditions effectively.

CHAPTER 7: THE WORLD OF GLUTEN-FREE BAKING

Gluten-Free Flours and Blends

Before diving into specific flour options, it's important to understand the role that gluten plays in traditional baking. Gluten is a protein found in wheat, rye, and barley that provides structure, elasticity, and chewiness to baked goods. Gluten-free flours lack this natural binding agent, which can result in dense, crumbly textures if not handled properly.

To achieve desired textures and consistency in gluten-free baking, it's often necessary to combine different flours or incorporate additional binding agents, such as xanthan gum, guar gum, or psyllium husk.

Single-Ingredient Gluten-Free Flours

Many gluten-free flours are made from a single ingredient, each offering its own unique flavor, texture, and nutritional profile. Here are some popular options:

1. **Almond Flour**: Made from finely ground almonds, this flour adds moisture, richness, and a nutty flavor to baked goods. It's high in protein, fiber, and healthy fats.

2. **Coconut Flour**: Derived from dried, ground coconut meat, this flour is highly absorbent and adds a subtle coconut flavor. It's rich in fiber and helps create a dense, moist texture.

3. **Rice Flour**: Available in both white and brown varieties, rice flour is mild in flavor and can be used for a variety of baked goods. It's a good source of carbohydrates and helps create a tender crumb.

4. **Oat Flour**: Made from finely ground oats, this flour adds a nutty flavor and helps create a tender, moist texture. It's a good source of fiber and often used in cookies, muffins, and quick breads.

5. **Buckwheat Flour**: Despite its name, buckwheat is not related to wheat and is naturally gluten-

free. It has an earthy, nutty flavor and is rich in fiber, protein, and minerals.

Gluten-Free Flour Blends

While single-ingredient flours can be used in certain recipes, many gluten-free bakers prefer to use pre-blended flour mixes for consistent results and improved texture. These blends typically combine various gluten-free flours with binding agents and starches to mimic the properties of wheat flour. Here are some popular options:

1. **All-Purpose Gluten-Free Flour Blends**: These versatile blends often include a combination of rice flour, tapioca starch, potato starch, and xanthan gum, making them suitable for a wide range of baked goods.

2. **Bread Flour Blends**: Formulated specifically for gluten-free bread baking, these blends often contain higher levels of protein and binding

agents to create a chewier, more bread-like texture.

3. **Whole Grain Blends**: For those seeking more nutrient-dense options, whole grain blends incorporate flours like sorghum, teff, and brown rice for added fiber and minerals.

4. **Gluten-Free Baking Mixes**: Many companies offer pre-measured, pre-blended mixes for specific baked goods like cakes, muffins, or pancakes, simplifying the gluten-free baking process.

When working with gluten-free flours and blends, it's important to follow recipes closely and experiment to find the combinations that suit your taste and texture preferences. Additionally, consider incorporating other gluten-free binding agents like chia seeds, flaxseeds, or applesauce to enhance moisture and structure.

Remember, gluten-free baking is an art and a science, and with the right ingredients and techniques, you can create delicious and satisfying gluten-free baked goods that rival their gluten-containing counterparts.

Mastering the Chemistry of Gluten-Free Baking

In traditional baking, gluten plays a crucial role in creating the desired structure, texture, and chewiness of baked goods. When flour is mixed with water and kneaded, the gluten proteins form an elastic network that traps air bubbles, allowing doughs and batters to rise and retain their shape during the baking process.

Without gluten, gluten-free doughs and batters lack this natural structure and tend to be dense, crumbly, and prone to spreading or collapsing during baking.

Binding Agents and Gums

To mimic the binding and structural properties of gluten, gluten-free bakers often rely on alternative ingredients known as binding agents or gums. These ingredients help to bind the flour and other dry ingredients together, creating a more cohesive and stable dough or batter. Some common binding agents used in gluten-free baking include:

1. **Xanthan Gum**: Derived from fermented bacteria, xanthan gum is a popular choice for gluten-free baking as it helps to bind ingredients, create structure, and trap air bubbles, resulting in a lighter, more bread-like texture.

2. **Guar Gum**: Similar to xanthan gum, guar gum is a plant-based thickener and binder that can improve the texture and stability of gluten-free baked goods.

3. **Psyllium Husk**: Ground psyllium husk, a soluble fiber derived from the Plantago plant, is an effective binder that can help create elasticity and chewiness in gluten-free breads and doughs.

4. **Chia Seeds and Flaxseeds**: These nutrient-dense seeds can be ground and used as natural binders in gluten-free baking, adding structure and moisture to baked goods.

It's important to note that binding agents should be used judiciously, as too much can result in a gummy or unpleasant texture.

Acid-Base Reactions and Leavening

In traditional baking, the combination of acidic and alkaline ingredients, along with the presence of gluten, creates a chemical reaction that helps doughs and batters rise and develop their desired texture. In gluten-free baking, alternative leavening agents and acid-base reactions must be employed to achieve similar results.

1. **Baking Soda and Acid Ingredients**: Baking soda, an alkaline ingredient, reacts with acidic ingredients like buttermilk, yogurt, or vinegar to produce carbon dioxide gas, which helps gluten-free batters rise and create a tender crumb.

2. **Baking Powder**: A combination of baking soda, an acid (usually cream of tartar), and a moisture-absorber, baking powder is a reliable leavening

agent for gluten-free baked goods, providing both rise and tenderness.

3. **Egg Whites**: Whipped egg whites can be incorporated into gluten-free batters to create a light and airy texture, mimicking the role of gluten in traditional baking.

4. **Yeast Breads**: For gluten-free bread baking, specialized bread flour blends and techniques, such as the use of psyllium husk or alternative binding agents, are often employed to create a chewy, bread-like texture.

Moisture Management and Fat Content

Gluten-free baked goods tend to have a shorter shelf life and can become dry or stale more quickly than their gluten-containing counterparts. Proper moisture management and the use of fats or oils can help to counteract this tendency.

1. **Fats and Oils**: Incorporating fats or oils, such as butter, coconut oil, or vegetable oil, can help to

improve the texture, tenderness, and moisture retention of gluten-free baked goods.

2. **Egg Yolks**: The lecithin in egg yolks can contribute to a richer, more tender crumb and improved moisture retention.

3. **Applesauce or Mashed Bananas**: These fruit-based ingredients can be used to replace some of the fat in recipes while adding natural moisture and binding properties.

4. **Dairy Products**: The addition of yogurt, sour cream, or milk can help to create a soft, moist texture in gluten-free baked goods.

Mastering the chemistry of gluten-free baking requires patience, experimentation, and a willingness to adapt recipes and techniques. By understanding the roles of binding agents, leavening agents, and moisture management, you can create gluten-free baked goods that not only satisfy dietary restrictions but also delight the senses with their texture, flavor, and appearance.

Remember, gluten-free baking is an ever-evolving field, and as new products and techniques emerge, the possibilities for delicious and innovative gluten-free creations continue to expand.

Baking Bread, Pastries, and Other Treats

Bread is often considered the holy grail of gluten-free baking, as it's notoriously difficult to replicate the chewy, elastic texture of traditional wheat-based loaves. However, with the right combination of gluten-free flours, binding agents, and leavening techniques, you can achieve remarkably satisfying gluten-free breads.

1. **Flour Blends**: Opt for specialized gluten-free bread flour blends that often include a combination of rice flour, tapioca starch, and xanthan gum or psyllium husk for improved structure and chewiness.

2. **Binding Agents**: Ingredients like psyllium husk, chia seeds, or flaxseeds can help create elasticity and bind the dough, mimicking the role of gluten.

3. **Leavening Techniques**: Experiment with different leavening agents, such as active dry yeast, sourdough starters, or a combination of baking soda and acidic ingredients, to achieve the desired rise and texture.

4. **Kneading and Proofing**: While gluten-free doughs may require less kneading than traditional bread doughs, proper kneading and proofing times are still crucial for developing flavor and structure.

5. **Enrichments**: Incorporate ingredients like eggs, milk, or butter to improve texture, moisture, and richness in your gluten-free breads.

Gluten-Free Pastries and Pies

Flaky pastries and pie crusts can be challenging to replicate without gluten, but with the right techniques and ingredients, you can create delightful gluten-free versions that will satisfy even the most discerning palates.

1. **Flour Blends**: Opt for gluten-free flour blends that include a combination of starches (such as tapioca or potato starch) and gluten-free flours (like rice flour or almond flour) to achieve a tender yet flaky texture.

2. **Cold Ingredients**: As in traditional pastry-making, using very cold butter, shortening, or alternative fats is essential for creating layers and flakiness.

3. **Binding Agents**: Xanthan gum or guar gum can help bind the dough and prevent crumbling.

4. **Egg Washes and Glazes**: Brushing your pastries with egg washes or glazes can help create a golden, shiny crust and improve browning.

5. **Blind Baking**: For pie crusts, blind baking (pre-baking the crust before adding the filling) can

help prevent sogginess and ensure a crisp, flaky texture.

Gluten-Free Cakes, Cookies, and Desserts

From decadent cakes to chewy cookies and indulgent desserts, the possibilities for gluten-free baking are endless. With the right flour blends, leavening agents, and binding ingredients, you can recreate your favorite sweet treats with ease.

1. **Flour Blends**: Look for gluten-free all-purpose flour blends or create your own blend using a combination of rice flour, almond flour, tapioca starch, and potato starch for optimal texture and structure.

2. **Leavening Agents**: Baking powder, baking soda, and whipped egg whites can help provide the necessary rise and airiness in gluten-free baked goods.

3. **Binding Agents**: Xanthan gum, guar gum, or ground chia or flaxseeds can help bind ingredients and prevent crumbling or spreading.

4. **Fats and Moisture**: Incorporate fats like butter, coconut oil, or applesauce to improve moisture retention and create a tender crumb.

5. **Flavor Boosters**: Don't be afraid to experiment with bold flavors, such as spices, extracts, citrus zests, or dried fruits, to enhance the taste and appeal of your gluten-free treats.

Remember, gluten-free baking is an art that requires patience, experimentation, and a willingness to adapt recipes and techniques. As you gain experience, you'll develop an intuition for the unique characteristics of gluten-free doughs and batters, allowing you to create truly remarkable baked goods that cater to your dietary needs without compromising on taste or texture.

Chapter 8: Family Matters: Going Gluten-Free with Loved Ones

Helping Your Family Adapt to Gluten-Free Cooking

Transitioning to a gluten-free lifestyle can be a significant adjustment, not just for the individual with dietary restrictions but also for the entire family. Whether you're navigating celiac disease, gluten sensitivity, or simply embracing a gluten-free lifestyle for personal reasons, ensuring that your loved ones are on board and equipped with the knowledge and skills to adapt to gluten-free cooking can make the journey smoother and more enjoyable for everyone involved.

Educating Your Family

The first step in helping your family adapt to gluten-free cooking is to educate them about the importance of adhering to a gluten-free diet. This can involve:

1. **Explaining Gluten and Its Effects**: Provide clear information on what gluten is, where it's found, and how it can impact individuals with celiac disease or gluten sensitivity.

2. **Highlighting the Benefits**: Discuss the potential health benefits of a gluten-free diet, such as improved digestion, increased energy levels, and reduced inflammation.

3. **Addressing Concerns**: Listen to your family's concerns or misconceptions about gluten-free living, and address them with factual information and empathy.

4. **Involving Children**: If you have children, involve them in the process by making it an educational and engaging experience, such as reading child-friendly books or watching videos about gluten-free living.

Creating a Gluten-Free Kitchen

To ensure a safe and allergen-free environment, it's crucial to establish a dedicated gluten-free kitchen area or take steps to minimize cross-contamination risks:

1. **Separate Cooking Utensils and Appliances**: Invest in separate sets of cooking utensils, pots, pans, and appliances (like toasters) that are used exclusively for gluten-free food preparation.

2. **Designate Gluten-Free Zones**: If sharing kitchen spaces, designate specific areas or surfaces as gluten-free zones to reduce the risk of cross-contamination.

3. **Proper Storage**: Store gluten-free products separately from gluten-containing items, and label them clearly to avoid confusion.

4. **Clean Thoroughly**: Implement a strict cleaning routine, using dedicated sponges and cleaning products to ensure surfaces are free from gluten residues.

Meal Planning and Grocery Shopping

Effective meal planning and grocery shopping strategies can make gluten-free cooking more manageable and enjoyable for the whole family:

1. **Involve the Family**: Invite family members to participate in meal planning and recipe selection, ensuring that everyone's preferences and dietary needs are considered.

2. **Plan Ahead**: Create a weekly or monthly meal plan that incorporates gluten-free options that the whole family can enjoy, reducing the stress of last-minute meal preparation.

3. **Read Labels Carefully**: Educate your family on how to read food labels and identify potential sources of gluten, such as hidden ingredients or cross-contamination risks.

4. **Stock Up on Gluten-Free Staples**: Keep your pantry and refrigerator stocked with gluten-free staples, like gluten-free flours, grains, pasta, and snacks, to make meal preparation easier.

Sharing Meals and Creating Traditions

Embracing gluten-free living doesn't mean sacrificing the joy and connection that comes from sharing meals and creating family traditions:

1. **Adapt Family Recipes**: Work together to adapt beloved family recipes to make them gluten-free, preserving the flavors and traditions that hold special meaning.

2. **Explore New Cuisines**: Use the transition to a gluten-free lifestyle as an opportunity to explore new cuisines and dishes that are naturally gluten-free or easily adaptable.

3. **Host Gluten-Free Gatherings**: Host gluten-free potlucks, dinner parties, or holiday gatherings, ensuring that everyone can enjoy the festivities without dietary restrictions.

4. **Create New Traditions**: Establish new family traditions around gluten-free cooking, such as hosting a monthly gluten-free baking night or

starting a gluten-free recipe exchange with friends and family.

Remember, adapting to a gluten-free lifestyle is a journey that requires patience, understanding, and a willingness to embrace change. By involving your family, educating them, and finding ways to make gluten-free cooking enjoyable and inclusive, you can foster a supportive and nurturing environment that celebrates the joy of food while prioritizing the health and well-being of every family member.

Gluten-Free Kids: Tips for Parents

A well-balanced, nutrient-dense diet is essential for a child's growth and development, and a gluten-free diet requires extra attention to ensure your child is receiving all the necessary vitamins, minerals, and other nutrients. Here are some tips to help you meet your child's nutritional needs:

1. **Focus on Whole Foods**: Emphasize whole, unprocessed foods like fruits, vegetables, lean proteins, gluten-free grains, and healthy fats to provide a wide range of essential nutrients.

2. **Supplement When Necessary**: Work with a pediatric dietitian or healthcare provider to identify any potential nutrient deficiencies and determine if supplements, such as iron, calcium, or vitamin D, are needed.

3. **Fortify Foods**: Incorporate gluten-free fortified foods, like cereals, breads, and pastas, to boost nutrient intake.

4. **Encourage Variety**: Introduce a diverse range of gluten-free foods to ensure your child is exposed to different flavors, textures, and nutrient profiles.

Promoting Healthy Habits

Instilling healthy habits from an early age can help your child develop a positive relationship with food and make gluten-free living a seamless part of their daily routine. Consider the following strategies:

1. **Involve Your Child**: Encourage your child's participation in meal planning, grocery shopping, and age-appropriate food preparation to foster a sense of ownership and understanding.

2. **Lead by Example**: Model healthy eating habits and a positive attitude towards gluten-free living, as children often mirror the behaviors of their parents and caregivers.

3. **Make it Fun**: Incorporate gluten-free cooking and baking activities into family time, making it an enjoyable and educational experience for your child.

4. **Celebrate Achievements**: Recognize and celebrate your child's efforts and achievements in adhering to a gluten-free diet, reinforcing positive behaviors and building confidence.

Social and Emotional Support

Living with dietary restrictions can be challenging for children, especially in social settings or when faced with peer pressure. Provide your child with the necessary support and coping strategies:

1. **Educate Others**: Work with teachers, caregivers, and other parents to ensure they understand your child's dietary needs and can provide a safe, inclusive environment.

2. **Teach Self-Advocacy**: Empower your child to confidently communicate their dietary requirements and make informed choices when eating away from home.

3. **Encourage Open Communication**: Create an open and supportive environment where your child feels comfortable discussing any concerns, challenges, or emotions related to their gluten-free lifestyle.

4. **Connect with Support Groups**: Join local or online support groups for parents of gluten-free

kids, where you can share experiences, seek advice, and foster a sense of community.

Navigating Special Occasions

Special occasions like birthdays, holidays, and social gatherings can present unique challenges for gluten-free kids. Prepare your child and ensure they can participate fully:

1. **Plan Ahead**: Contact hosts or venues in advance to discuss gluten-free options and make necessary accommodations.

2. **Bring Gluten-Free Alternatives**: Pack gluten-free snacks, treats, or a safe meal option for your child to enjoy, ensuring they don't feel left out.

3. **Educate and Advocate**: Politely educate others about your child's dietary needs and advocate for their inclusion in activities and celebrations.

4. **Create New Traditions**: Establish new family traditions that are naturally gluten-free or easily

adaptable, fostering a sense of inclusivity and joy.

Raising a gluten-free child requires patience, diligence, and a commitment to creating a supportive and nurturing environment. By prioritizing your child's health, promoting healthy habits, and fostering their confidence and self-advocacy skills, you can help them navigate the gluten-free lifestyle with ease and empower them to thrive in all aspects of their life.

Planning Gluten-Free Meals Everyone Will Enjoy

Transitioning to a gluten-free lifestyle can be a daunting task, especially when catering to the diverse dietary needs and preferences of an entire family. However, with a little creativity and strategic planning, you can create delicious and satisfying gluten-free meals that everyone at the table will enjoy, regardless of their dietary restrictions.

Embrace Naturally Gluten-Free Foods

One of the easiest ways to plan gluten-free meals that appeal to the whole family is to emphasize naturally gluten-free foods. These are foods that are inherently free from gluten and don't require extensive modifications or substitutions. Some examples include:

Fresh fruits and vegetables: A wide variety of fresh produce, from crisp salads to roasted veggies, can form the basis of flavorful and nutrient-dense gluten-free meals.

Lean proteins: Grilled or baked meats, poultry, fish, and eggs are naturally gluten-free and can be prepared in countless delicious ways.

Nuts and seeds: Incorporate nutrient-rich nuts, seeds, and nut butters into your meals for added texture, flavor, and healthy fats.

Gluten-free grains and starches: Quinoa, rice, corn, potatoes, and gluten-free oats offer versatile and satisfying options for gluten-free meals.

By focusing on these whole, unprocessed foods, you can create balanced and flavorful meals that cater to various dietary needs without sacrificing taste or nutrition.

Adapt Family Favorites

Instead of completely overhauling your family's favorite recipes, consider adapting them to be gluten-free. This approach can make the transition smoother for everyone, as familiar flavors and dishes remain on the table while accommodating dietary restrictions.

Substitute gluten-free flours: Replace wheat flour with gluten-free alternatives like rice flour, almond flour, or gluten-free all-purpose flour blends in baked goods and breaded dishes.

Explore gluten-free alternatives: Opt for gluten-free pastas, breads, and crackers to replace their gluten-containing counterparts in traditional recipes.

Get creative with seasonings and sauces: Experiment with bold spices, herbs, and flavorful sauces to enhance the taste of gluten-free dishes and compensate for any textural differences.

Involve the family: Encourage family members to share their favorite recipes and work together to adapt them, ensuring that everyone's preferences are considered and celebrated.

By making slight adjustments to beloved family recipes, you can maintain cherished traditions while ensuring that everyone at the table can enjoy the meal safely and without compromise.

Meal Planning Strategies

Effective meal planning can streamline the process of creating gluten-free meals that appeal to the whole family. Here are some strategies to consider:

Plan ahead: Develop a weekly or monthly meal plan that incorporates a variety of gluten-free options, allowing you to shop and prepare efficiently.

Batch cook and repurpose leftovers: Cook larger portions of gluten-free staples, like grains, proteins, and sauces, and repurpose them in creative ways throughout the week for easy, flavorful meals.

Embrace one-pot or sheet-pan meals: These versatile cooking methods allow you to prepare entire meals with minimal effort, while accommodating different dietary needs with personalized portions or toppings.

Include family favorites: Incorporate family-friendly gluten-free dishes, like tacos, stir-fries, or pasta dishes made with gluten-free alternatives, to ensure everyone feels satisfied and included.

By planning ahead and employing efficient cooking techniques, you can streamline the process of preparing gluten-free meals that cater to the diverse preferences of your family members.

Remember, the key to successful gluten-free meal planning is to focus on fresh, whole foods, adapt beloved family recipes, and involve your loved ones in the process. With a little creativity and an open mind, you can create delicious, nutritious, and inclusive meals that bring everyone together around the table, regardless of their dietary needs.

CHAPTER 9: ADVANCED GLUTEN-FREE LIVING

Staying Gluten-Free During Travel

Proper planning is essential for a successful gluten-free travel experience. Here are some steps to take before you depart:

1. **Research Your Destination**: Investigate the availability of gluten-free dining options, grocery stores, and local cuisine that naturally accommodates a gluten-free diet at your destination. Online forums, travel guides, and local celiac associations can be valuable resources.

2. **Notify Travel Providers**: When booking accommodations or transportation, inform the relevant providers of your dietary requirements. Many airlines, hotels, and cruise lines offer

gluten-free meal options or can make special arrangements upon request.

3. **Pack Gluten-Free Essentials**: Stock up on gluten-free snacks, protein bars, and non-perishable items to have on hand during travel and in case safe options are limited at your destination.

4. **Prepare Translation Cards**: If traveling to a country where you don't speak the language fluently, prepare translation cards or a mobile app that explains your dietary needs in the local language.

5. **Equip Your Travel Kit**: Pack essential items like a portable gluten-free kitchen kit (including utensils, condiments, and a small cooler), food storage containers, and cleaning supplies to maintain a gluten-free environment on the go.

Dining Out and Accommodations

Navigating dining options and accommodations while traveling can be challenging, but with the right strategies, you can enjoy a seamless gluten-free experience:

1. **Research Restaurants**: Before your trip, research gluten-free-friendly restaurants at your destination or look for establishments that cater to dietary restrictions. Online reviews and gluten-free dining apps can be invaluable resources.

2. **Communicate Clearly**: When dining out, clearly communicate your dietary needs to servers or chefs. Don't be afraid to ask questions about ingredients, preparation methods, and cross-contamination protocols.

3. **Choose Accommodations Wisely**: Consider staying at accommodations with kitchen facilities, allowing you to prepare your own gluten-free meals. Alternatively, look for hotels or resorts that offer dedicated gluten-free menus

or have experience catering to special dietary needs.

4. **Be Prepared for Emergencies**: Keep a stash of gluten-free snacks or emergency rations in case safe dining options are unavailable, especially during long flights, road trips, or remote destinations.

Cultural Awareness and Exploration

Embracing local cuisines and traditions can be a highlight of any travel experience, and with a little creativity, you can enjoy the flavors of your destination while staying true to your gluten-free diet:

1. **Explore Naturally Gluten-Free Cuisines**: Many traditional cuisines, such as Indian, Mexican, and Mediterranean, feature naturally gluten-free dishes or can be easily adapted to accommodate your dietary needs.

2. **Seek Out Local Markets**: Visit local farmers' markets, specialty food stores, or outdoor

markets to source fresh, naturally gluten-free ingredients and experience the authentic flavors of your destination.

3. **Attend Cooking Classes**: Participate in gluten-free cooking classes or food tours to learn about local ingredients and preparation techniques that align with your dietary requirements.

4. **Connect with the Local Community**: Reach out to local celiac associations or gluten-free support groups for insider tips, recommendations, and a deeper understanding of navigating a gluten-free lifestyle in your travel destination.

Staying gluten-free while traveling requires diligence, preparation, and a willingness to adapt and explore. By researching your destination, communicating your needs, and embracing local culinary traditions, you can enjoy a safe, satisfying, and enriching travel experience without compromising your dietary requirements.

Embrace the adventure and savor the flavors of the world, one gluten-free bite at a time.

Preparing for Holidays and Special Occasions
Planning and Communication

Effective planning and open communication are key to ensuring a seamless and stress-free gluten-free experience during holidays and special occasions. Consider the following strategies:

1. **Discuss Dietary Needs**: If you're attending a gathering at someone else's home, have an open and honest conversation with the host about your gluten-free requirements. Offer to bring a dish or two to ensure you have safe options.

2. **Coordinate with Family and Friends**: For family gatherings, involve your loved ones in the planning process. Discuss menu options, ingredient lists, and cross-contamination concerns to ensure everyone is on the same page.

3. **Research Restaurants and Venues**: If celebrating at a restaurant or event venue, research their gluten-free offerings and policies in advance. Don't hesitate to call ahead and discuss your dietary needs with the staff.

4. **Plan Ahead for Travel**: If your holiday plans involve travel, prepare accordingly by packing gluten-free snacks, researching dining options at your destination, and communicating your needs with airlines, hotels, or other travel providers.

Navigating Shared Meals and Potlucks

Shared meals and potlucks can be a minefield for those following a gluten-free diet, but with the right strategies, you can participate fully and safely:

1. **Bring Your Own Dish**: Prepare a gluten-free dish or two that you know you can enjoy without worry. Consider making extra portions to share with others who may also have dietary restrictions.

2. **Label Your Dishes**: Clearly label your gluten-free dishes to avoid confusion and cross-contamination. Consider using separate serving utensils and containers to further minimize risks.

3. **Educate Others**: Take the opportunity to educate family and friends about your gluten-free needs and the importance of avoiding cross-contamination. Share reliable resources or enlist their help in keeping surfaces and utensils separate.

4. **Be Mindful of Cross-Contamination**: Pay close attention to shared serving utensils, cutting boards, and preparation surfaces to avoid accidental exposure to gluten. Don't be afraid to politely inquire about ingredients or preparation methods.

Gluten-Free Entertaining and Hosting

If you're hosting a holiday gathering or special occasion, you have the opportunity to create a safe and inclusive environment for your gluten-free guests. Here are some tips to consider:

1. **Plan a Gluten-Free Menu**: Design a menu that is entirely gluten-free or offers ample gluten-free options. Consider traditional dishes that can be easily adapted or explore new gluten-free recipes.

2. **Create a Dedicated Preparation Area**: Set up a dedicated gluten-free preparation area in your kitchen to minimize the risk of cross-contamination. Use separate utensils, cutting boards, and cookware for gluten-free items.

3. **Label and Identify Gluten-Free Dishes**: Clearly label all gluten-free dishes and provide ingredient lists or allergen information to help guests make informed choices.

4. **Accommodate Special Diets**: Be mindful of guests with multiple dietary restrictions, such as those who are gluten-free and vegan or dairy-

free. Offer a variety of options to cater to different needs.

5. **Provide Gluten-Free Beverages and Desserts**: Don't forget to offer gluten-free beverage options and indulgent gluten-free desserts to ensure everyone can fully participate in the celebrations.

Remember, holidays and special occasions are meant to be enjoyed by all. By planning ahead, communicating openly, and taking the necessary precautions, you can create a safe, inclusive, and memorable experience for yourself and your loved ones, regardless of dietary restrictions.

Advocating for Gluten-Free Options in Schools and Workplaces

Advocating in Schools

Education plays a crucial role in shaping the future, and ensuring that gluten-free students have access to safe and nutritious meals is paramount for their academic success and overall well-being. Consider the following approaches when advocating for gluten-free options in schools:

1. **Educate School Staff**: Schedule meetings with school administrators, food service staff, and teachers to provide comprehensive education on celiac disease, gluten sensitivity, and the importance of maintaining a gluten-free diet. Share reliable resources and offer to collaborate on training efforts.

2. **Propose Gluten-Free Menu Options**: Work with the school's food service department to develop a gluten-free menu that offers a variety of nutritious and appealing options. Suggest incorporating naturally gluten-free items, as well as gluten-free alternatives for popular dishes.

3. **Encourage Safe Food Handling Practices**: Advocate for the implementation of strict food handling protocols to prevent cross-

contamination, such as dedicated preparation areas, utensils, and storage containers for gluten-free items.

4. **Support Inclusive Classroom Policies**: Collaborate with teachers and school administrators to establish policies that ensure gluten-free students can participate fully in classroom activities, field trips, and special events without compromising their dietary needs.

5. **Form a Parent Support Group**: Connect with other parents of gluten-free students to create a support network and collectively advocate for change within the school system. Strength in numbers can amplify your voice and drive meaningful change.

Advocating in Workplaces

Maintaining a gluten-free lifestyle should not compromise an individual's professional growth or workplace experience. By advocating for gluten-free options in the workplace, you can create an inclusive and supportive environment that promotes employee well-being and productivity. Consider the following strategies:

1. **Educate Human Resources and Management**: Schedule meetings with human resources professionals and management to discuss the importance of accommodating gluten-free employees. Provide resources and offer to collaborate on developing inclusive policies and practices.

2. **Propose Gluten-Free Options in the Cafeteria or Breakroom**: Work with the food service provider or facility management to introduce gluten-free options in the cafeteria or breakroom. Suggest dedicated gluten-free sections, clear labeling, and cross-contamination prevention measures.

3. **Encourage Inclusive Workplace Events and Meetings**: Advocate for the inclusion of gluten-free options during workplace events, meetings, or catered functions. Offer to assist in menu planning or provide recommendations for gluten-free caterers or vendors.

4. **Support Workplace Wellness Initiatives**: Collaborate with human resources or wellness committees to promote gluten-free awareness and education as part of workplace wellness initiatives. Offer to host workshops, seminars, or informational sessions on living a gluten-free lifestyle.

5. **Connect with Colleagues**: Reach out to other gluten-free colleagues or employees with dietary restrictions to form a support network. Together, you can advocate for change and raise awareness within the organization.

Advocating for gluten-free options in schools and workplaces requires persistence, education, and collaboration. By working closely with stakeholders, providing reliable resources, and offering practical solutions, you can create environments that prioritize the health and well-being of individuals with celiac disease or gluten sensitivity. Remember, your advocacy efforts not only benefit those with dietary restrictions but also promote inclusivity, understanding, and a sense of community for all.

CHAPTER 10: LOOKING AHEAD: THE FUTURE OF GLUTEN-FREE

Advancements in Gluten-Free Product Development

The gluten-free market has witnessed significant growth and innovation in recent years, and this trend is expected to continue as consumer demand and technological advancements drive product development:

1. **Improved Taste and Texture**: As research and development in gluten-free food technology progresses, we can expect to see gluten-free products that more closely mimic the taste, texture, and mouthfeel of their gluten-containing counterparts.

2. **Expansion of Gluten-Free Options**: With increasing awareness and demand, we'll likely see a broader range of gluten-free products

available in mainstream grocery stores, restaurants, and food service establishments, making it easier for individuals with celiac disease or gluten sensitivity to navigate dining experiences.

3. **Nutrient-Dense Formulations**: As the focus on health and wellness continues to grow, gluten-free product developers may prioritize the incorporation of nutrient-dense ingredients, such as ancient grains, superfoods, and functional additives, to enhance the nutritional value of gluten-free offerings.

4. **Sustainable and Ethical Sourcing**: With increasing consumer interest in sustainable and ethical practices, we may see a greater emphasis on sourcing gluten-free ingredients from responsible and environmentally friendly sources, as well as a focus on fair trade and ethical labor practices.

Advancements in Medical Research and Diagnosis

The medical community's understanding of celiac disease and gluten-related disorders is continually evolving, and advancements in research and diagnostic techniques may reshape the way these conditions are identified and managed:

1. **Improved Diagnostic Tools**: Researchers are exploring new and more accurate methods for diagnosing celiac disease and non-celiac gluten sensitivity, potentially leading to earlier and more reliable diagnoses.

2. **Personalized Treatment Approaches**: As our understanding of the genetic and environmental factors contributing to gluten-related disorders deepens, we may see the development of personalized treatment approaches tailored to an individual's specific needs and circumstances.

3. **Alternative Therapies**: While a strict gluten-free diet remains the primary treatment for celiac

disease, researchers are investigating potential alternative or complementary therapies, such as enzyme supplementation or immunotherapy, that could provide additional options for managing the condition.

4. **Increased Awareness and Education**: With continued research and increased public awareness, we may see improved education and training for healthcare professionals, leading to better recognition, diagnosis, and management of gluten-related disorders.

Societal and Cultural Shifts

As gluten-free living becomes more mainstream, we may witness broader societal and cultural shifts that contribute to greater inclusivity and acceptance:

1. **Increased Mainstream Acceptance**: As more individuals embrace gluten-free living for various reasons, we may see a continued normalization of gluten-free diets, leading to

greater understanding and accommodation in social and cultural settings.

2. **Improved Labeling and Regulations**: With growing consumer demand and advocacy efforts, we may see stricter labeling regulations and better enforcement of gluten-free claims, providing greater transparency and confidence for consumers.

3. **Inclusive Dining Experiences**: Restaurants, event venues, and food service establishments may continue to prioritize inclusive dining experiences, offering dedicated gluten-free menus, trained staff, and strict protocols to prevent cross-contamination.

4. **Increased Representation and Advocacy**: As the gluten-free community continues to grow and organize, we may witness increased representation and advocacy efforts, leading to greater awareness, support, and policy changes

that benefit individuals with celiac disease and gluten sensitivity.

The future of gluten-free living holds immense promise, with exciting developments on the horizon across various sectors. From advancements in product development and medical research to societal shifts and increased inclusivity, the gluten-free landscape is poised for positive change. As we look ahead, it's crucial to stay informed, support ongoing research, and continue advocating for the needs and well-being of those following a gluten-free lifestyle. By embracing these changes and working together, we can create a future where living gluten-free is not only a necessity but a celebrated and widely accepted way of life.